The Mineral Magnesium

"An informational course in nutrition to help you prevent and eliminate disease"

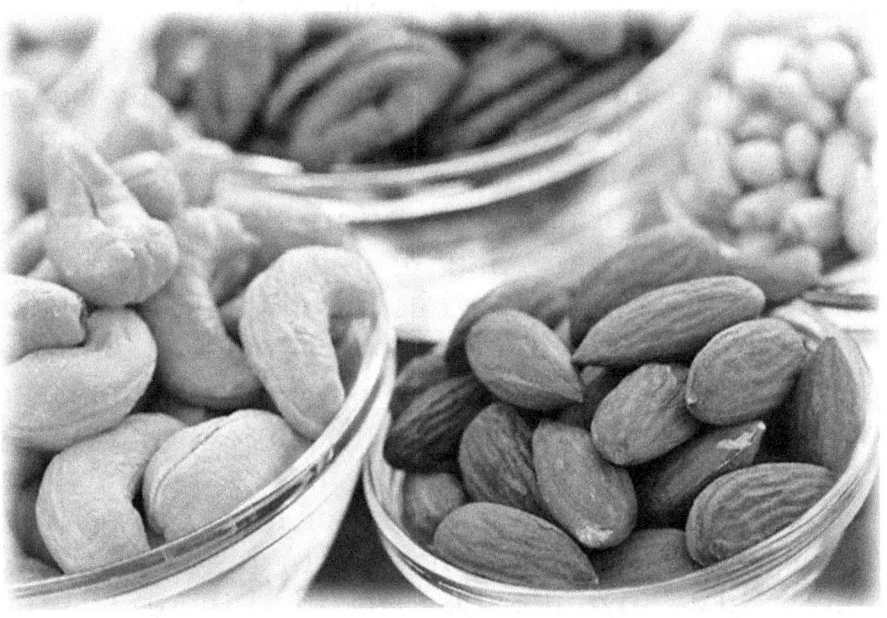

Rudy S Silva, Natural Nutritionist

Best Nutrition Diet: The Mineral Magnesium © 2012 by Rudy S Silva

ISBN-13: 978-1492967927
ISBN-10: 1492967920

First Printing, 2012 Printed in the United States of America

Table of Contents

Chapter 1: Introduction

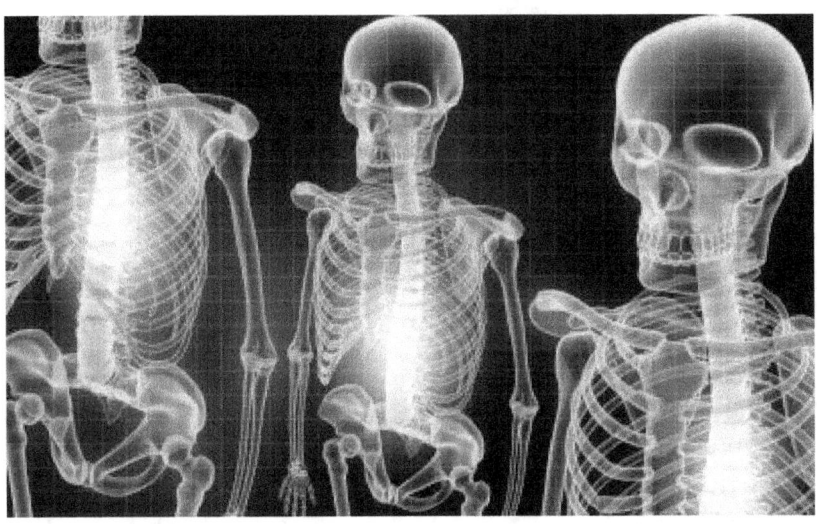

Half of the magnesium you have in your body is found in your bones, and the other half is in your soft tissue. It is found in your skeletal muscles, liver, heart and pancreas.

Magnesium is considered a "forgotten mineral." Most people don't think about magnesium like they do calcium, potassium or iron. Almost 90% of the population may be short on magnesium, since it has been found that they only consume about 40% of the daily recommended requirement.

If you are short in magnesium, you may not show any symptoms, you may just ignore them, or you may attribute them to some other nutrient deficiency. However, moderate or severe magnesium deficiency results in malnutrition, loss of appetite, nausea, weakness, personality changes and arrhythmias.

Magnesium in Chlorophyll

Magnesium is a major mineral like sodium, calcium, and potassium. It is central to the food chain in that it holds a position in chlorophyll, the blood of plants. It appears in the center of the chlorophyll molecule. Chlorophyll is similar to the hemoglobin molecule except that at the center of the hemoglobin molecule is the mineral iron.

So, if you want to build your blood, drinking chlorophyll is one ways to do. It's the magnesium in the chlorophyll that also helps make white blood cells that fight infection and, which combines with red blood cells.

When your body is low in hemoglobin, drinking chlorophyll will help increase the hemoglobin in your blood. Your body has the power to transmute or to transform magnesium into iron, which helps to make more hemoglobin. It does this through multiple chemical changes that start with oxygen.

Magnesium Requirements

The overall balance of minerals in your body's lymph liquids, outside your cells and inside your cells, determines your health. When your minerals are balanced similar to sea water, you will have better health.

The sea has a high level of magnesium, so that water inside your cells should also be high in magnesium, since magnesium is used to transport nutrients in and out of your cells. Magnesium is a major mineral that is needed in the right quantities, so that you can achieve maximum health.

Most people ignore the importance of magnesium. It is important to know what magnesium does in your body. You need to know what foods to eat to get the maximum magnesium in your body. You should know what symptoms you will have, when you don't get the proper amount of magnesium.

If you know how magnesium is regulated in your body, then you can help your body maintain and keep the amount that your body needs. Also, if you know what illnesses need more magnesium, you can help yourself get well.

Magnesium and Enzymes

Magnesium is involved in activating over 300 different enzymes and body chemicals. It helps to active the B vitamins. It works in protein synthesis, muscle excitability and helps to release energy. In your cells, it converts fat, carbohydrates, and protein into the energy your body needs. It helps to regulate blood sugar, nerve impulses, and electrical potential across cell walls. And, it tones brain blood vessels and keeps them relaxed and open, so that nutrients can get into your brain cells.

Magnesium and Bones

You will find magnesium, mostly in your cells, in the mitochondria, which is the energy center of your cells. Magnesium regulated the absorption of calcium and maintains the construction of bones and teeth. Lack of magnesium can lead to brittle bones and osteoporosis. Your parathyroid gland also needs magnesium to regulate your blood calcium levels.

Magnesium is the third most important nutrient in building bones, after calcium and vitamin D. Half of all the magnesium in your body is found in your bones. When you lack magnesium, you are susceptible to forming calcium crystals in your bones and in other body locations.

Stress

If you are constantly under stress because of your job, your home life, or your regular life, then most likely, you will be low on magnesium. The same holds true if you stress your body physically by doing exercise and playing sports.

Chapter 2: The Magic of the Mineral Magnesium

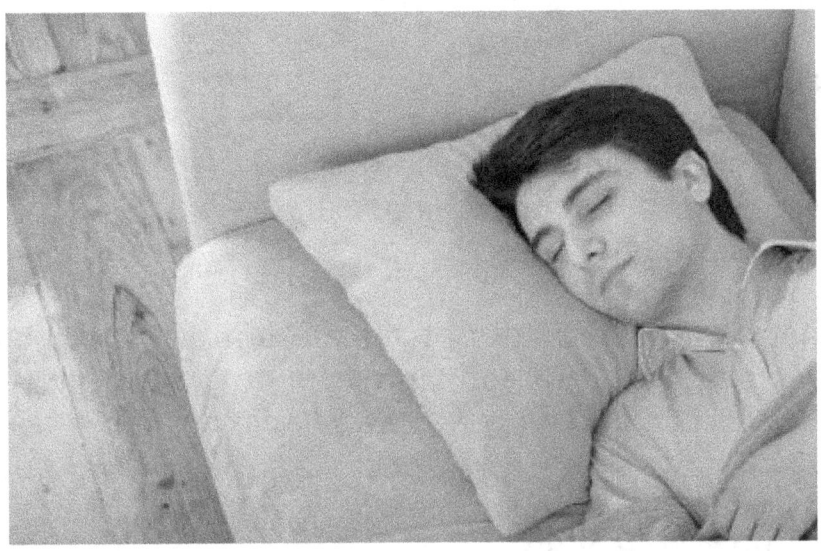

"A mineral that relaxes the body – magnesium"

Like **sodium**, calcium, and **potassium**, magnesium also has a positive charge and is represented by the symbol, Mn+. Because of this, magnesium helps to make your body more alkaline. Your bones hold up to 60% of the body's magnesium, and the extracellular liquid contains around 1%.

Your body holds up to 3 oz. of magnesium. It is alkaline in nature and it is known as the "Relaxer", since helps to calm the nerves and muscle tissue. But, calming your nerves is also a matter of mind control and attitude. You can increase your life span, when you are calmer and have the proper amount of magnesium in your body.

In your body, magnesium takes the form of:

Magnesium carbonate
Magnesium silicate
Magnesium chloride
Magnesium sulphate (Epsom salt)
Magnesium phosphate.

When you have plenty of magnesium in your body, you have good motion and can do many physical activities. Here is a list of what magnesium does in your   body.

Alkalinizes the body
Produces laxative action
Calms the nerves
Keeps the body flexibly
Influences glands
Combats acids and toxins
Eliminates poisons
Prevents deposition of phosphates in joints
Neutralizes phosphoric acid
Promotes carbohydrate metabolism in the cells
Helps produce and use body energy
Helps in DNA and protein creation
Assists Potassium and sodium cross-cell membrane during Potassium – Sodium Pump action
Regulates muscle movements

Helps maintain calcium levels in the extracellular fluid

Magnesium does its work by reducing tension, relaxing your body, and improving bowel movements. It reduces nerve irritation by neutralizing the chemicals or by-products that are created when your body is going through tense and irritable conditions.

Your body regulates the amount of magnesium it retains and stores by using the gastrointestinal tract, GI tract, and urinary system. If you need more magnesium in your body, the GI tract will absorb more in the small intestine. If your body has too much magnesium, the GI tract will excrete some of it and eliminate it through your stools.

Your kidneys are also involved in controlling the amount of magnesium your body retains. If magnesium levels fall, the kidneys closely control how much magnesium goes into your urine. Similarly, if the magnesium levels are too high, the kidneys will excrete more through your urine.

Regulation of Magnesium

Many things control how much magnesium and calcium you absorb. If magnesium in your body goes up, calcium stores will go down and if magnesium stores fall, then calcium body stores go up. Your stomach absorbs a lot of magnesium for hydrochloric acid production, HCl. When you take in food or calcium supplements, protein, vitamin D, or alcohol, your body needs more magnesium. And, caffeine, sugar, phosphorus, excess sodium, diuretics, and alcohol increase the loss of magnesium through urine.

You will increase the amount of magnesium you absorb, when you drink milk, because of the presence of lactose.

Magnesium as a laxative

Magnesium has natural laxative powers. When you eat foods that have magnesium your regularity improves. When magnesium is consumed and reaches your blood, some of it is transported into your colon walls. Where, it softens your stools and helps to produce peristaltic action. For this reason fruits and vegetables that contain some or are high in magnesium promote regularity – yellow and winter squashes, grapefruits, apricots, oranges, peaches, and corn.

Chapter 3: Foods That Give You The Best Magnesium

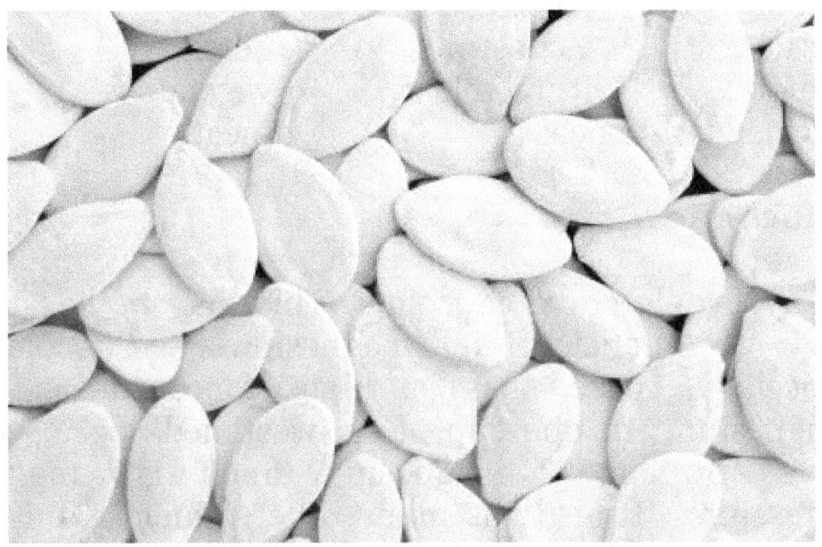

Here is a list of the foods that you should eat to get plenty of magnesium:

Best foods with magnesium:

Rice bran, pumpkin seeds, wheat germ, sunflower seeds, sesame seeds, seaweed agar, cashews, hazelnuts, fermented soy products

Other great foods for magnesium:

Peanuts	leafy greens	seeds
Buckwheat	bananas	beet greens

Oats	avocados	black-eyed peas
Baked potato	with skins	blackstrap
molasses		
Cabbage,	dandelion	brown rice
Rice bran,	pomegranates	barley
Whole wheat	walnuts	mustard greens
Almonds	nuts	rye
Nettles	chestnuts	berries
Seafood	green leafy	vegetables
Dry beans and peas		meat

Chocolate

Many people crave chocolate. This may be because they are deficient in magnesium. Chocolate, especially cocoa, has a high concentration of magnesium. In one cup of unsweetened cocoa, you have 400 mg of magnesium and 2159 mg of potassium. It also has many other minerals, but in smaller quantity. Cocoa is also known for is high level of antioxidants.
To get the best benefits of cocoa, you need to eat chocolate that has at least 85% cocoa.

However, when you eat chocolate candy, which has bittersweet chocolate, or semisweet baking chocolate, it has up to 65% sugar and a fat level of 20 – 35%. Cocoa has 2% sugar and has a fat level of up to 15%. Using unsweetened or bittersweet chocolate in cooking is ok, since its sugar level is 2 – 45%.

What is not good about chocolate is it is also high in caffeine and theobromine, which stimulate the adrenals that can lead to adrenal fatigue.

Yellow Cornmeal

Yellow cornmeal, high in magnesium, has excellent laxative powers. Use it 3 or 4 times a week and improve your regularity. Cornmeal, cooked slowly under low heat, can easily be used with children or adults who are constipated. Or, you can prepare raw corn soup by:

- 1 ½ cups raw corn off the cob

- Vegetable broth to taste

- 2 bay leaves

- 1 ½ cup of raw milk, cream, or milk

- Put all this into a blender and warm slightly

Calms the nerves

Magnesium is a relaxer of nerves. When you are tense, nervous, get irritated, or turn hot tempered, you develop ulcers, colitis, constipation, and colon spastic conditions. Magnesium will help to reduce or minimize these conditions. It enters the nerve fibers, with the help of albumin and water.

When you first take magnesium for nerves or for any other condition, you will have to use it for a month or more to see results. It takes that long and even longer for magnesium to fill your body reserves, so that it is available to serve your body's needs.

If you have lower-back problems, you need to have plenty of magnesium. When you are tense, any adjustments a chiropractor gives will go out of adjustment, when your body is low in magnesium. The adjustment will be made, and your tense ligaments or muscles will pull back the adjustment to its previous position. Magnesium is found in tendons, ligaments, tissue, joints, and nerves and helps them to relax and to maintain bones in position.

Night cramps in your calves call for magnesium and calcium, which prevents the stiffening of tissue and muscle due to excess acids.

Alkalizes the body

Magnesium combines with acids, gases, waste, impurities, and toxins to clean your body and make your body more alkaline.

Magnesium sulphate pulls toxic buildup and waste from your intestinal walls and eliminates them through your stools.

A good supply of magnesium is necessary to make your body alkaline and to combine with poisons and heavy metals. Magnesium can combine with poisons that create diseases. It combines with excess albumin, lead, phosphorus, chloride, antimony, 'ferrous sulphate, barium, muriatic acid, uric acid, urate acid, and ptomaine.

In the brain, magnesium combines with phosphoric by-products that occur when you do excessive mental work.

Chapter 4: Conditions Caused By Excess or Deficient Magnesium

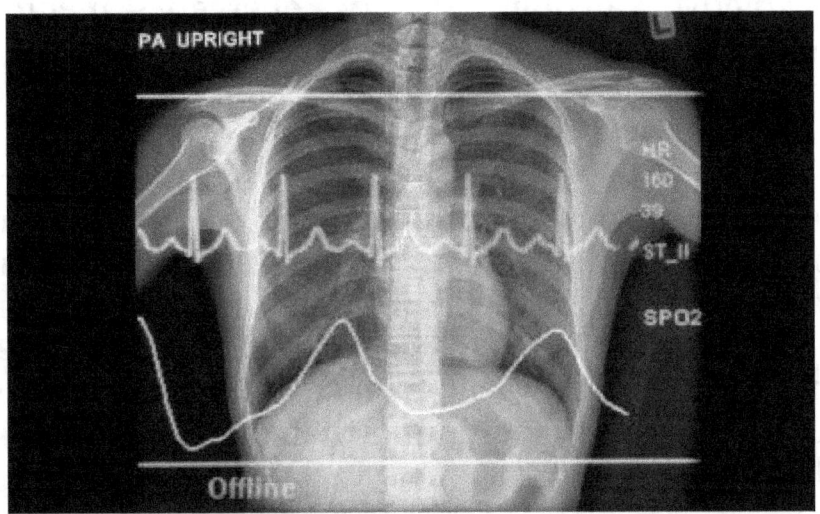

Deficiencies of Magnesium

When you become dehydrated, you lose magnesium. When you take calcium, you will deplete your stores of magnesium. Drinking too much milk also will deplete your body's magnesium.

Young athletes who drink too much milk need to be careful, since they tend to lose magnesium. Retired and geriatric people should always take a magnesium supplement.

If you are taking diuretics of any kind, natural

remedies or drugs, you will slowly lose your magnesium. The more diuretics you use the more magnesium you lose.

When you are deficient in magnesium, you are over sensitive about everything in your life. You are hyperactive, anxious, fidgety, energetic, mentally active, and industrious. There are so many symptoms when you are deficient in magnesium that it is hard to tell when you are deficient.

The more serious symptoms are muscle spasms and seizures. There is now some evidence that magnesium deficiency has an important role in many heart ailments. Dr. Alexander Heggtveit, at the University of Ottawa in Canada, found fatal attack victims with less magnesium than those that died of other causes.

You can have a magnesium deficiency after prolonged diarrhea and vomiting or with long term laxative and diuretic use. If you frequently drink too much alcohol then, you will be deficient in magnesium.

Elderly people are at high risk for magnesium deficiency, since they absorb it poorly. If they supplement with too much calcium or use too many drugs, this can deplete their magnesium body stores.

When you have a low level of magnesium, you will have an increase in calcium blood levels, which contribute to the formation of kidney stones. If the low levels continue, magnesium will be pulled out of the heart muscles, causing a disruption in its function.

When your blood levels of magnesium are low, your body takes magnesium that is stored in your tissues, which leads to muscle weakness, fatigue, irritability and nervousness.

Here is a list of symptoms you can have when you have a low level of magnesium.

- Head tremors
- Voice breaks or stammers
- Unclear conversations
- Feeling of doom
- Smelly feet
- Muscles are weak
- Constipation
- Poor kidney function
- Poor sleep
- Back pain
- Heart palpitations
- Eyelids twitch
- Osteoporosis
- High blood pressure
- Migraine headaches
- Appetite for acid food and drink
- Nausea
- Heavy head in morning
- Shoulder and neck muscles tense at night

Hypomagnesemia

A deficiency in magnesium is called Hypomagnesemia. This deficiency is when the amount of your body's magnesium falls below 1.8mEq/L. The unit mEq/L is a measure given to the amount of substance in a body per liter. This deficiency can occur when you:

- don't eat enough magnesium foods

- have poor absorption of magnesium in GI tract

- have excess magnesium loss in GI tract

- have excess magnesium loss in urinary tract – kidney

- use excess coffee, alcohol, sugar, and tobacco

Negative emotions also deplete magnesium that is in reserves and in intracellular liquid. If you constantly live these emotions below, then you will be short of magnesium:

Hatred, resentment, jealousy, quarrels, bitterness, temper outbursts, selfishness, greed fear, panic, worry, paranoia, overwork, over study, loss of love one.

Other symptoms you can have with low magnesium are:

- Cardiac arrhythmias
- Digoxin toxicity
- Laryngeal strid or Respiratory muscle weakness
- Seizures
- Arthritis deformans
- Poor elimination
- Over excitement
- Nervous headaches
- Ulcers
- Acute diarrhea
- Eyes tearing excessively or excess catarrh of eye lens
- Nosebleeds
- Sex brain nerve ends and nerve fiber irritation
- Decrease in electrical nerve impulse
- Extreme colitis
- Urine retention
- Sleeplessness, fainting
- Hot temper, forgetfulness
- Drastic mood changes
- Increase in asthmatic attacks
- Free-Radical Damage

When you are magnesium deficient, the body starts taking magnesium out of your cells. As you reduce cell magnesium, your muscles grow weak and nerves and muscles become highly irritable.

Free-Radical Damage

Low levels of magnesium can magnify the damage caused by free radicals. It has also been seen that it can start the production of free radicals.

Excess of Magnesium

You can have excess magnesium in your body, when you eat an excess of magnesium foods, supplements, tonics or drugs. When you have an excess of magnesium in your body, the sedative effects of magnesium are intensified. What happens is that your memory decreases, you become less active, and do not have good reasoning skills. Your nerve endings become less sensitive and depressed, and your perception and intelligence is decreased. You become less interested in life and you sleep more.

Hypermagnesemia

Excessive magnesium in your body is called Hypermagnesemia. This condition occurs when you have a magnesium level above 2.5 mEq/L. This condition is rare, since kidneys can quickly remove excess magnesium. But, when it does occur, and the cause could be:

- Kidney dysfunction
- Addison's disease
- Adrenocortical insufficiency
- Excess use of antacids or laxatives
- Excess use of magnesium rich dialysate
- Excess use of TPN solutions

- Excess use of magnesium sulfate in treating seizures, or hypertension

Patellar Reflex

If your patellar reflex, the tapping just below the knee to see if the leg extension occurs, is absent, it's an indication that your magnesium level is 7 mEq/L or higher. This high level makes your nerves relax creating an absence of leg reflex in the patellar test.

Magnesium Laxative

Excess magnesium is quickly removed, from your body by the onset of diarrhea. But, one of the issues is that you can develop an excess of magnesium when you use a large amount over-the-counter, drugstore products, for acid reflux or constipation. Overdose on magnesium is a rare occurrence.

Large amounts of magnesium can be toxic. You can end up with excess magnesium, if you have kidney disease or if your calcium body levels are low and your phosphorus intake is high.

Chapter 5: Magnesium Supplements And Natural Remedies

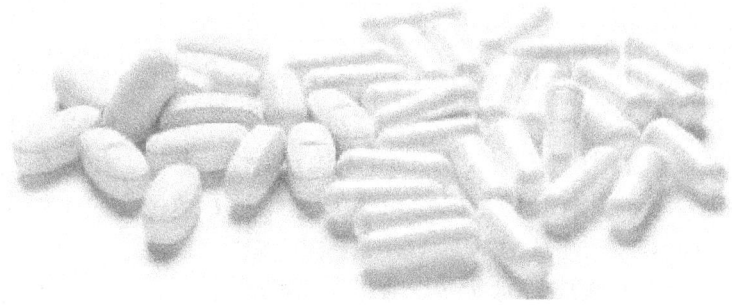

Taking Magnesium Supplements

Do not take magnesium supplements if you have kidney weakness or disease. Also, if you have heart problems, do not take more than 350 mg of magnesium. It is always safe to see your doctor about what dose you should take.

Fast Magnesium

If you have gut spasms or other body conditions where you need to receive magnesium fast, you can do it as follows:

Buy a Magnesium Chloride Solution 18%, Ecologic Formulas Brand, on the Internet or at a health-food store. Add 1-2 teaspoons to a glass of water and drink twice a day. The taste is not too good, but you will get magnesium into your body quickly.

It is estimated that a typical American diet provides only around 30% to 50% of the 500 mg of the daily requirements for magnesium. In addition, around 80% of the diets eaten in American are magnesium deficient.

Magnesium is easier to lose than other minerals and especially when you eat or take an increase in calcium. When you supplement with magnesium, you should check that the supplement has equal amounts of magnesium and calcium. If it has more calcium, you will lose some magnesium. Or, it would be better to take magnesium as a separate supplement and taken when you don't take calcium.

Magnesium Citrate

Use a magnesium citrate supplement. Take this supplement after 8pm with vitamin C and pantothenic acid, since these three nutrients work together. Always take magnesium and all other minerals and trace minerals with tomato juice or apple juice or at meals with whole grapes, meat or digestive enzymes. This provides acid to dissolve and absorb the magnesium quicker. You can also take it after 8pm or just before bedtime without any food.
.

There are other forms of magnesium that are also good, since they are tied to an amino acid or are so called "chelated."

- Magnesium citrate

- Magnesium gluconate,

- Magnesium Aspartate

- Magnesium taurate

- Magnesium oxide – avoid using this type, because it is not as absorbable as the other types.

Magnesium and Calcium Supplements

Look for a combination supplement of calcium, magnesium,
vitamin D and with a 1:1 ratio of calcium to magnesium. This type of ratio is hard to find, but you should be able to find it on the Internet. Most ratios your will find are 2:1 with calcium being twice as much as magnesium.

Here are other some other magnesium combinations that you should consider, if you can't fine the supplements above:

Potassium- magnesium citrate
Magnesium citrate – potassium- taurine

Taking too much magnesium can cause diarrhea, lethargy or weakness. This mineral can also interfere with any antibiotic you might be taking, so it best not to supplement with it when taking antibiotics or even other drugs.

How Much Magnesium?

Some doctors and nutritionists say that, you should have twice as much magnesium as calcium in your supplement. This will ensure that you will have strong bones. Most supplements that contain these minerals are of the opposite ratio; they have twice as much calcium as magnesium. But, taking a supplement with a 1:1 ratio should be where you can start.

Daily magnesium supplementation is:

- Children to 14 years, 270 mg

- Males 15 and older, 500 mg

- Males 51 years and older 600 mg

- Females 15 and older, 300 mg

- Females 51 years and older 550 mg

In some cases for adults up to 1200 mg is recommended. Over dosing is very hard with magnesium, since the kidney and the colon will excrete the excess. If you start to exhibit signs of diarrhea or body weakness, back off on the amount you are taking.

Vitamin D

You need the proper levels of magnesium to activate the vitamin D your body needs. If you have a magnesium deficiency, then you will have lower levels of vitamin D. Make sure you have the Vitamin D3 type of supplement.

B vitamins

When you take Vitamin B6, you improve the intake of magnesium into your cells. You can supplement with a vitamin B 50 or 100 to get the needed B vitamins.

Copper

Because magnesium is easily lost in the urine, when you are dehydrated, you can take 3 mg of copper, and this will stop the loss of magnesium in your urine.

Over The Counter Magnesium Products

Magnesium toxicity can occur with individuals with kidney failure. Toxicity effects have been found in some individuals that use laxative such as Epsom salts, magnesium sulfate and milk of magnesia, or magnesium hydroxide. These laxatives are typically used at 3,000 to 5,000 mg per day. Toxic effects have been found when these laxatives are used at 9,000 mg per day.

If you have a deficiency of magnesium, it will take around 6 months of magnesium supplementation to get your body back to normal levels of magnesium. Your body uses magnesium every day, so you need to supply it with this amount every day. Any excess can go to neutralize acids. Then if still have some left over, this will go to various body areas to be store.

Chapter 6: Illnesses that You Cure With Magnesium

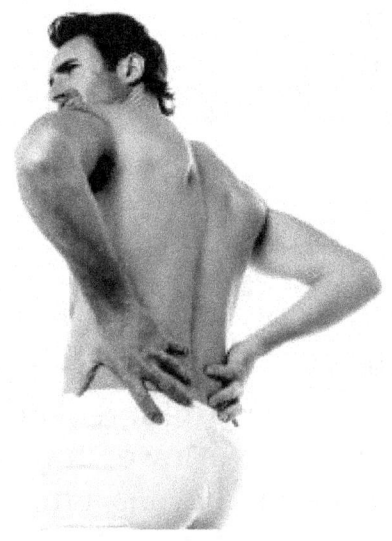

There are certain illnesses that you can reduce, eliminate and even cure, if you increase your intake of magnesium. Some of these illnesses are caused by the lack of magnesium.

These illnesses are:

- Cardiovascular
- Chronic fatigue syndrome
- Kidney stones
- Muscle cramps
- Preeclampsia – during pregnancy

- Osteoporosis
- PMS symptoms
- Migraines
- Respiratory disease
- Alzheimer's disease
- Back problems
- Free Radicals
- Migraines
- Digestive Problems
- Eye problems
- Constipation

Cardiovascular

Having a low level of magnesium can result in more blood clots. It has been found that women that use oral contraceptives have lower levels of magnesium. This is the reason why there is a higher occurrence of thrombosis in women who use these contraceptives.

A deficiency of magnesium can damage the arteries in the heart, which results in plaque buildup. High blood pressure is also associated with a magnesium deficiency. There is a tendency for those with diabetes and low magnesium to have more cardiovascular issues.

So keep your levels of magnesium high by eating and supplementing with the suggestions given here. Magnesium helps to reduce the possibility of you having a heart attack, stroke, angina, or heart surgery. Eating nuts of various kinds every work day will help you stop heart attacks.

Kidney Stones

If you have kidney stones, you can get rid of them by using 1000 mg of magnesium citrate and 100 mg of B6. If you just want to make sure you don't accumulate stones, you can use this supplement combination on occasion for a week. Kidney stones are a combination of calcium and oxalic acid. When these two combine in the kidney, they form calcium oxalate crystals. To minimize the amount of oxalic acid you have in your body, avoid eating cooked spinach or other green tops. Eat them raw when possible.

Muscle Cramps

Magnesium helps to relax muscle and without it, you are prone to muscle cramps. When calcium moves into muscle tissue, your muscles will contract. When calcium leaves the muscles, and magnesium moves into your muscles, your muscles will relax. Excess deficiency of magnesium leads to muscle spasms, tremors, and convulsions. If you have leg cramps at night, take a combination of calcium, magnesium, and vitamin D. This will put an end to these cramps. Take this supplement just before bedtime.

Osteoporosis

To have strong bones and teeth you need minerals. It's calcium that makes bones strong in conjunction with other minerals such as phosphorous, magnesium, strontium, silica, zinc, copper, and boron. Magnesium is definitely needed to prevent osteoporosis.

PMS symptoms

There are some women who crave chocolate before their period or who have PMS. It is known that magnesium helps resolve the symptoms of PMS, since it is involved in the production of progesterone. A lack of magnesium can produce decreased progesterone levels resulting in PMS symptoms.

It's better to avoid chocolate, since it creates adrenal fatigue. It is better to eat those foods that are high in magnesium or to take 400 mg of magnesium citrate. Take this magnesium with some vitamin C and B6 just before bedtime. Magnesium is absorbed better after 8pm. This combination of nutrients will help to reduce the intensity and duration of PMS.

Pregnancy

Magnesium has a powerful influence in the prevention of pregnancy complication, such as prematurity and intrauterine growth retardation.

Migraines

There are studies that show magnesium can prevent or relieve migraines. By using high doses of 1000 mg or more, magnesium was shown to be just as effective as established drugs, such as flunarizine and amitriptyline.

Respiratory Disease

Magnesium is helpful in respiratory disease such as bronchitis and asthma. Eat those foods that are high in magnesium, but you need to be aware of those foods that you might be allergic to, which aggravate your respiratory condition.

Alzheimer's Disease

Having a low level of magnesium and calcium in your body opens you up to toxic aluminum deposit in your brain nerve cells. When you have these low levels of these minerals, your body will accept the use of other minerals in their place. So if you also have an excess of aluminum, your body will use it in place of magnesium or calcium and when these minerals reach your brain, they deposit in your brain cells.

The result is that you have the onset of senility, or you develop Alzheimer's. Under these conditions, zinc is the recommend mineral to prevent senile changes in your brain.

Magnesium is involved in keeping your brain cells alive. It does this by reducing the negative effects of less blood flow to the brain and by insuring that nutrients reach your brain cells. It also prevents the buildup of calcium in your brain cells, which is associated with Alzheimer's.

Back Problems

Magnesium will help you build a strong straight back. It aids in the inter-vertebral structure. It is in this structure where magnesium is stored. It is also stored in the colon. If the vertebral structure and colon don't get enough magnesium, they will not function properly.

Free Radicals

It has been seen by researchers that low levels of magnesium give way to free-radical formation thus exposing cells to more radical attack.

Migraines

It has been found that 50% of people with migraines have magnesium deficiency. You can get some relief by taking 400+ mg of magnesium daily with meals.

Digestive Problems

If you have stomach problems such as vomiting, cramps, indigestion, flatulence, stomach pain, or constipation, all this could be related to low levels of magnesium.

Eye problems

If you are diabetic, you will want to keep high levels of blood magnesium. If you do, you are less likely to develop diabetic retinopathy. In addition, if you have glaucoma, it will lessen the effects of this condition.

Constipation

Magnesium is hydrophilic and likes water. In your colon, it will draw water and make your stools soft. Magnesium is used in many over-the-counter laxatives. Using these laxatives, gives you high levels of magnesium salts. If you are deficient in magnesium, you will have constipation.

Sweaty Hands

Have you ever shaked hands with someone who has sweaty hands or that has excess body order? Aside from not showering frequently, this person may be deficient in magnesium. The use of liquid chlorophyll will help reduce the body order.

Chapter 7: Final Comments

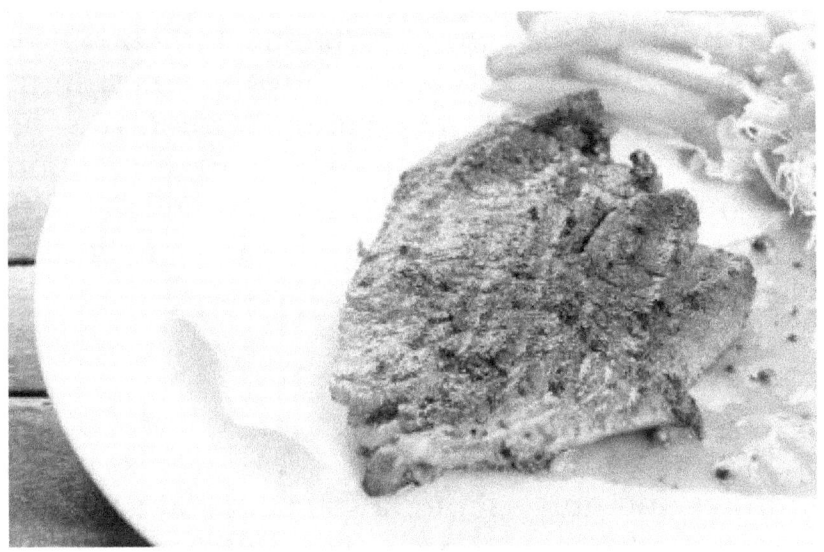

In your cells, tissues, muscles, and nerves, magnesium neutralizes acids, toxic matter, and wastes that are created when you become anxious, nervous, hot tempered, over excited, or overworked. It helps to neutralize those acids that come from eating too much acid food. Use magnesium foods and supplements to help get your body alkaline.

When you eat a lot of meat and other acid foods with little vegetables, you will deplete your stores of magnesium, and you will need to use all the information listed in this book to restore your magnesium body levels.

Magnesium is known as the "Relaxer" since it calms your nervous and muscular system.

You can have an under or over supply of magnesium in your body. Your kidney and colon are responsible for maintaining the proper magnesium balance in your body. It will excrete excessive magnesium into your urine, or it will stop excreting it when your body supplies are low. And, with under supplies, magnesium will be pulled out of your cells to satisfy your body's needs. When it does this your body will be acidic and prone to disease.

Eat Magnesium Foods

Eat magnesium foods daily. Use seeds in your smoothies and nuts as midday snacks. Eat a variety of vegetables. Choosing 4 or 5 vegetable properly can give you plenty of all the minerals you need. However, by choosing a variety of fruits and vegetables, you get certain nutrients and antioxidants that are only available in each fruit or vegetable.

Magnesium Supplements

When you buy a magnesium supplement, it is best to buy it with calcium and vitamin D. Calcium needs magnesium and vitamin D to complete its digestion and absorption into your body. Choose those supplements that are tied to an amino acid, like Magnesium Citrate. This allows this mineral to be pulled through your intestinal wall easier and faster. Look for a magnesium supplement that has just as much magnesium as calcium, 1:1.

If you have a lot of anxiety and stress in your life, you will need to take up to 1000 mg of magnesium. Stress uses up a lot of magnesium.

Look at the list of illnesses and body conditions listed in the previous chapters and see if you have some of these symptoms or diseases. If so, then you too should be taking up to 1000 mg of magnesium. If you have issues with your kidney or heart, then talk to your doctor about how much magnesium you should take.

Excess Magnesium

If you take too much magnesium, you will get diarrhea. Just back off on the amount you are taking, until your diarrhea goes away.

Chapter 8: About The Author And Other Resources

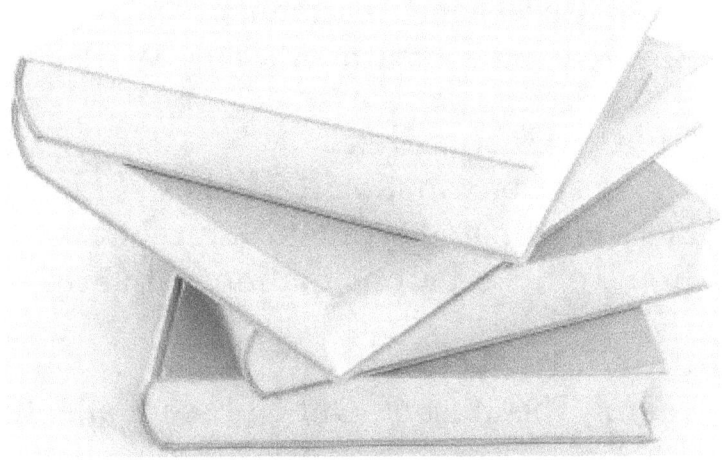

Get one of my best kindle books *free* below:

http://www.natural-remedies-thatwork.com

Rudy Silva is a natural nutritional consultant educated in the United States in Nutrition and Physics.   He is a graduate from San Jose State University in California. He is author of 45 other books on natural remedies.   He has authored a newsletter in natural remedies for over 10 years.

Resource page

Here are some of the other kindle e-books about natural remedies that have been written by this author. You can see the entire list at:

http://tinyurl.com/b2f7wd3

Acne Remedies
- Best natural acne treatments: Acne facial
- Effective Acne Treatments That Work

Constipation Remedies
- The Best Constipation Remedies
- Best Constipated Women Natural Cures
- How To Relieve Constipation With Fruits

Essential Fatty Acids
- Taking The Mystery Out Of Essential Fatty acids
- Amazing Fish Oil Benefits Revealed
- Omega 3 and 6 Mystery Exposed

Nutrition Remedies
- Updated Version - Secret Diet And Nutrition
- Secret Healthy Fruit Practices Revealed
- Fast Healing Juice Nutrition Therapy: Nutrition Tips 3
- Fantastic Alkaline Fruit Benefits Revealed
- Calcium (Discover How To Use Calcium To Avoid Devastating Diseases)
- Magnesium Nutrition Revealed

- Best Nutrition Health Practices
- Potassium Health Secrets Revealed
- Phosphorus, The Best Brain Food
- A Sodium Diet (What You Must Know About Sodium)
- Vegetables and Vegetable Juice Cures
- Alkaline Body: How to Change an Acid Body into an Alkaline body

Stomach Remedies

- Acid Reflux: Fast and Easy Cures For Acid Reflux
- Asthma Treatment Cures With Remedies
- How To Do Natural Colon Cleansing
- Gastrointestinal Digestion Secrets Revealed

Misc Remedies

- Natural Hair Loss Treatment: Women And Men
- Effective Natural Hemorrhoids Treatment
- Iron Deficiency Anemia
- Secrets To Understanding Behavior
- Fast Acting Ear Infection Remedies
- Best Behavior Secrets Revealed That Can Change Your Personality
- What Is A Hiatus Hernia
- Best Varicose Vein Treatments?
- Make Shampoos At Home Using Natural Ingredients:Discover recipes for quality natural hair shampoos
- How To Fix Your Thyroid Problems: Discover Hidden Ideas That Fix Your Thyroid

Minerals

- Calcium and Magnesium Magic Body Benefits Revealed
- The Magic of Sodium, Calcium and Magnesium
- Create an Alkaline Body with Potassium and Sodium: Eliminate a Potassium Deficiency
- Calcium and Phosphorus Foods: Deficiency or Excesses in These Minerals Cause Bone and Brain Power Loss
- Chlorine The Body Detoxifier (With water, chlorine will clean your body of toxins and pathogens)

Men's Health

- Best Impotence Health Diet

Weight loss

- Ten (10) Day Quick Success Weight Loss Program: A new approach to losing weight by changing your eating habits for life
- Discover Secret Anti-Aging Juice & Tonic Recipes: Unique Juices And Tonics That Create Beauty And Youth

To see all the kindle books written by this author, go to this the Authors Profile Page or this URL:

http://tinyurl.com/b2f7wd3

If you need support or want to promote any of his e-books, please contact him at rss41@yahoo.com and expect a reply within 24 hours. He looks forward to hearing from you and is happy to help you understand his material on natural and nutritional health.

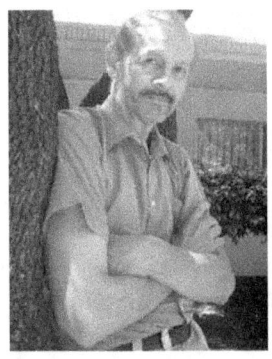

Give A Review

And, don't for get to give a review for this e-book at Amazon so that others can gain the benefits of what is in this e-book. To you, for losing weight, creating better health and more happiness in your life,

Rudy S Silva

www.ingramcontent.com/pod-product-compliance
Lightning Source LLC
Chambersburg PA
CBHW070838290526
45795CB00002B/910